CW01497538

Running for Weight Loss

A Guide on Running for a Healthier and Thinner You

Sam Hignett

CONTENTS

Introduction

If you're looking for a fun way to lose some weight without the need for a faddy diet then choosing to run is a great first step on the way to your goals.

I have been running for many years but before I started I tried to lose weight using many different diets and training programs. Nothing ever seemed to work and if it did it was only briefly and I was soon putting on the weight again.

When I took up running a few things happened almost straight away that kept me motivated and I haven't looked back since.

First of all and most importantly it was easy and fun. There was no expensive gym membership or equipment to buy. Secondly I found that the post run buzz, even after just a few short runs, made me feel great and improved my self esteem almost immediately. Third and finally I discovered that even after a few short weeks the weight was falling off me and I was feeling great. The compounding effect of these three immense transitions to my wellbeing meant I haven't stop running since and this was over 15 years ago!

So thanks for purchasing this book and I hope that you too will soon be noticing the differences running can make to your life.

Thanks and good luck!

Chapter 1 – Nutrition

Nutrition is one of the most important building blocks in maintaining a healthy lifestyle. But what is it exactly?

Nutrition can be described very simply. It is supplying our body with the nutrients it needs to maintain a healthy, balanced system and to supplement growth (in the case of children). The main source of these nutrients is the foods we eat.

But therein lies a problem, in today's modern world many of us are eating incorrectly and this has sent obesity rates, in both adults and children, skyrocketing.

Why are humans getting bigger?

There are a number of reasons why mankind is steadily getting bigger. Figures in the United States show that obesity rates have tripled since the 1980's.

- We are eating more junk food and eating more calories

  This simple fact means we are consuming far more calories than we used to. Junk food is processed and extremely high in calories. It is low in fibre (which keeps us feeling full) as well as high in sugar and saturated fats. Simply put, junk food makes your blood sugar levels spike extremely quickly, leaving you feeling hungry in an hour or so after you have eaten it.

- We are consuming more sugar than ever before

Much like with junk food, sugar consumption has also increased. There are many reasons for this, but the main cause is linked to the junk food we consume – it is filled with sugar. Consuming too much sugar affects our metabolism. In some people, this can lead to a number of conditions including insulin resistance, fat gain around the belly and raised bad cholesterol (LDL) levels. Excessive sugar consumption can also lead to type 2 diabetes.

- We are consuming more sugary drinks and fruit juice than ever before

The human brain is an amazing organ, but it has some faults. Our brains help to control our energy balance, making sure we don't starve and also that we don't consume too much food either.

It has a slight fault, however. It does not see liquid sugar calories in the same way that it sees calories gained from regular food. When we drink a sugary drink, our brain lets this by, not calculating it into our daily intake and therefore not regulating our bodies into eating fewer calories.

Soft drinks are filled with sugar, but another major culprit are fruit juices. People think that because fruit is a healthy option, fruit juice is fine as well. It isn't. Fruit should be consumed in its raw state, never as a liquid. If you prefer fruit juice over fruit, rather dilute it with water and limit yourself to one glass a day.

- We are consuming more food as there is such a variety available

Studies have shown that the more food varieties we have available to eat, the more food we end up eating. Just think about it. Have you ever been to a buffet? Don't you end up trying a little bit of everything? You eat more than is necessary don't you?

- We burn fewer calories than ever before.

Today we live a much more sedentary lifestyle than 50 years ago. Many modern professions, especially office based ones, are not as physically demanding as those of generations before us. In those times, a large number of people did not live in the city. They did, however, perform physically demanding jobs that burnt more calories than our jobs today.

- We consume more vegetable oil than ever before.

With the rise in consumption of both junk and processed food, we are ingesting far more vegetable oil than previous generations. Vegetable oil is extremely high in calories.

- We sleep less than ever before.

Sleep is a very important part of our daily routine. Our body needs it. A lack of sleep often leads to weight gain as it can affect certain hormones in our body. These hormones, ghrelin and leptin, are directly responsible for controlling our appetites. Studies have shown that adults who do not get enough sleep are 55% more likely to gain weight.

- Stress related comfort eating

  We live in a very fast-paced, stressful world. Often people deal with their stress through comfort eating, usually consuming junk food. Unfortunately, this leads to weight gain.

- Aggressive marketing

  Companies that sell fast foods spend millions on advertising, often with false claims about their products. This marketing and advertising works, if it didn't, they wouldn't spend the money!

Chapter 2 – Why Running?

Running is one of the most popular exercises in the world. Millions of runners take to the streets, parks and trails every day, running mile after mile. But why do they do it?

There are a many reasons to take up running. Let's take a look at them in more detail.

Running benefits your health

Running is one of the best ways to improve your fitness, and through that, your health. By running, your body is benefited in the following ways:

- Running increases lung capacity

  Lung capacity is often overlooked when it comes to determining a person's physical condition as more emphasis is placed on heart health. The truth is, as a person gets older their lung capacity begins to diminish. In fact, by the age of 50, a person's lung capacity has shrunk by up to 50% compared to their early 20's.

  How exactly does this affect your health? Well, a smaller lung capacity means that less oxygen travels in your blood around your body and into cells. Less lung capacity also leads to many conditions that include shortness of breath, less endurance and leaves people more at risk to respiratory illness. Other negative factors from decrease lung capacity include a lower metabolic function, a higher risk of both strokes and heart attacks, lowered energy levels, fatigue, memory loss and concentration problems.

Studies have shown that exercise, especially high-intensity exercises such as running, can increase lung capacity over a period of time. This is achieved by creating an oxygen debt in the lungs, activating certain metabolic processes that cause their capacity to increase.

- Running raises the levels of good cholesterol in your body

Studies have shown that regular, high-intensity exercise such as running (30 minutes, 5 times per week) can boost your HDL (good) cholesterol levels by as much as 5% when compared to people who lead a more restful existence.

- Running can help to boost your immune system

By exercising, your body gets stronger in a number of ways. Firstly, your heart strengthens and with that its ability to pump blood and oxygen through your body improves. Secondly, exercise strengthens your muscles. Thirdly, exercise will help to augment the cells in your body, especially those that fight off bacteria that cause infections or sickness.

- Running can help to prevent blood clots

Studies have shown that high-intensity exercise such as running can help to reduce the chances of blood clots occurring. It does this by causing platelets to be less "sticky". Platelets in the blood are tasked with forming clots when bleeding occurs, although sometimes they can clot together in the blood stream, especially during periods of extended inactivity such as long distance travel.

Running can help to prevent disease

Another positive aspect of running is that it can help to prevent numerous diseases.

- Breast cancer

  Studies over the past number of years have shown that regular exercise can help reduce breast cancer by up to 25%. Although scientists do not yet fully understand how this happens, it is thought that exercise helps to control various hormones in the body, including oestrogen. Higher levels of this hormone can lead to the onset of breast cancer.

- High blood pressure

  As mentioned earlier, exercising helps to strengthen the heart, which is essentially a muscle. This, in turn, means the heart can operate more effectively, pumping blood around the body with ease. This effectively lowers blood pressure, but this does not happen overnight. You will have to exercise for between 1 to 3 months to reap the benefits.

- Diabetes

  Many studies from all over the medical fraternity have shown that exercise can fight the onset of type-2 diabetes. For people who are already diabetic, exercise helps muscles in the body to consume more glucose. This lowers our blood glucose, keeping it at acceptable levels. Exercise also stops blood glucose levels from spiking after meals, a problem for most diabetics.

Running can help to relieve stress

In today's modern world, stress is something we cannot escape. It is often brushed off by those suffering from it, but it can cause major health problems and mood swings. There are various ways people can deal with it however, and running is an excellent outlet. Exercise can help to lower our fatigue levels, make us more alert as well as give us the ability to concentrate better. It also raises our endorphin levels which leads to better rest and, therefore, reduced stress.

Running can help to fight depression and anxiety

People who suffer from depression and anxiety are often told to exercise to help fight their conditions. Depression acts on the brain in various negative ways but especially by slowing down its ability to create dopamine, norepinephrine and serotonin, all known mood enhancers.

Exercise can help fight this as it produces proteins that force the brain to start creating mood enhancers once again.

Running can help to lose weight

Running is one of the best ways to burn calories and lose weight. There are many reasons for this.

- Afterburn

  An exercise undertaken at high-intensity helps the body to continue to burn calories long after it has ended. This is known as the "afterburn". Although all exercise can generate this effect, high-intensity training means it happens for longer periods after the session is finished. This promotes more efficient weight loss. Studies have shown that running is 90% more effective when it comes to weight loss than walking or other low-intensity exercises.

- Burns fat

  A high intensity running session is a great way to target fat and burn it off. For instance, run at a normal pace for 60 seconds, and then run as fast as you can for 30 seconds. Rest for 60 seconds and repeat. Running up hills also is a great way to specifically target fat.

- Time-efficiency

  Running is a very time-efficient exercise, capable of burning more calories more quickly than other low-intensity exercises.

- Convenient

  Running is one of the easiest exercises to start. The only thing you need is a decent pair of running shoes and little else, except maybe a little bit of willpower. You can run anywhere and at any time... and it's cheap!

Other benefits of running

Running can:

- Strengthen bones.
- Help with joint flexibility.
- Improve circulation.
- Help with insomnia.

Chapter 3 – Let' s get started! A guide to running equipment

Running, luckily, is not a sport that needs tons and tons of equipment. You will need a decent pair of shoes, and proper running attire. There are some other useful accessories that you can consider adding to your equipment at a later date.

Perhaps the most important piece of equipment that you will require is your shoes. Without the correct shoes, your running career will be over before it gets off the ground!

Choosing the correct shoes. How do you pronate?

Let's begin by looking at something called pronation.

What is pronation? Well, every runner's feet strike the ground very differently when they run. Pronation is how the runner's foot rolls inward as they take each stride. This movement takes place in the subtalar joint found just below the ankle. It is broken down into two types; under pronation or overpronation. Determining your pronation characteristics goes a long way towards selecting running shoes that will work for you.

Why do our feet pronate as we run? Well, for a number of reasons. Firstly, pronation takes the shock of the first contact with the ground. So basically, it acts as a shock absorber. Secondly, pronation helps our feet and brains to determine the kind of surface that the runner is on. It then automatically adjusts and stabilizes each foot to the terrain type.

- Neutral pronation

  A runner with neutral pronation will strike the ground near the centre of their foot. This allows for a wide variety of running shoe options.

- Underpronation

  When runners underpronate, the outside of their heel hits the ground first, followed by the rest of the outside of their feet. Most of the wear on the shoe will be on the outside of the foot. Runners who underpronate are very susceptible to stress fractures and, therefore, require running shoes with a very specific cushion on the outer half of the shoe.

- Overpronation

  When a runner overpronates, their heel strikes the ground but then rolls with an inward motion. All weight is placed on the inside portion of the feet and not the ball of the foot. Ultimately, this causes instability as the foot of the runner always has to counterbalance against movement inwards. This leads to injuries, especially to the hips and knees. Runners who overpronate need shoes that provide excellent support and cushioning on the inner half of the shoe.

Now you probably have a fair idea the type of pronation that affects your feet. If you don't, here is a quick and easy test to help you.

- Wet the sole of your right foot.
- Stand on a brown paper bag or something where your foot will leave an imprint.
- Study the imprint left behind.
- If around half of your arch is visible, then you are a normal pronator.
- If much of your arch is showing, you overpronate.
- If very little of your arch is showing, you underpronate.

Although you should be going to a running store to determine the best running shoe for your pronation type, here is a very basic guideline that you can follow.

- Normal pronation running shoes

  As a normal pronator, you can wear a wide range of running shoes. Try, however, to purchase shoes that give stability especially medial stability. Moderate arch support is important as well.

- Overpronation running shoes

  As an overpronator, you will need running shoes with built-in support such as dual-density midsoles. Other, more expensive options such as motion-control running shoes give the best support and are needed if the overpronator is tall, heavy or run with a bow-legged style.

- Underpronation running shoes

   As an underpronator, you will need running with a neutral cushioning pattern with soft midsoles. This encourages the foot to fall in a more natural manner.

Please note, this is just a very basic guideline to the running shoes that the various pronation styles should use. When buying your shoes, you should consult directly with an expert at a running store. In this way, you will go a long way to preventing unnecessary injuries by ensuring you have the correct shoes.

Choosing the correct shoes. The importance of the correct size.

Although this is a very simple suggestion, often people do not buy the correct size shoes. All shoes are different. You might think that your feet are a particular size, but always try on a running shoe before purchasing it. Another suggestion, wear both shoes for a period in store to see how it feels on your feet. The wrong size shoe will only lead to injuries.

- Here are a few important things to consider regarding the correct size shoe.
- As we get older, our feet get larger. Just because you wore a size 8 the last time you ran ten years ago doesn't mean your feet are the same size now.
- In general, a running shoe will be a half a size bigger than your regular shoes.

- If you do make an error, it is better to run in a shoe that is slightly too big than a shoe that is too small.
- When trying a running shoe, use the same socks that you would use while you run.
- Rather go shopping for running shoes in the afternoon than in the morning. As the day wears on, our feet swell. This is especially important if you will be running in the evening when your feet are at their largest.

Once you have found the perfect running shoe and have tried them on, make sure they fit correctly by taking note of the following.

- Firstly, your heel should fit fairly tightly into the back of the shoe. It should never slip upwards.
- Secondly, the mid-section of your foot (under your arch and over the instep of your foot) should also fit securely into the shoe. This should not be too tight, however.
- Thirdly, you should be able to wiggle your toes at the front of the shoe. Remember, as your feet strike the ground, they will move forward slightly, so there needs to be some room for them to move. Your feet will also swell as you run. Leave a gap of around the width of a thumbnail between your biggest toe and the shoe's front.
- Fourthly, note the width of the shoe in relation to the width of your foot. The shoe should be fairly tight towards the back, becoming less fitted as your move forward along your foot. If the material is very tight near the ball of your foot you will need a wider shoe.

Choosing the correct shoes. The importance of flexibility.

The importance of a running shoe's flexibility cannot be emphasised enough, this is often overlooked, however.

When we run, our feet flex. For this very reason, we need a running shoe that flexes in more or less the same position that our feet do, particularly when it comes to the area around the balls of our feet.

Luckily, there is a simple test that can quickly determine if a shoe is flexing in the correct position. Here is what you need to do. Take a running shoe and hold it tightly near the heel. Now bend the shoe upwards from the front, near where your toes would be. Observe where the shoe flexes. If it flexes near the middle, start looking for another shoe. The flex should happen near where the ball of your feet would be.

Of course, as with many things in life, there can be exceptions. Some runners suffer from pain in the balls of their feet, especially when they flex upwards. If this is the case, getting a running shoe that flexes more to the middle would be appropriate.

Flexibility comes in another form. It is important also to check how much the shoe can twist on it's Y-axis. This is important, as you want a shoe that doesn't flex too much in this way as to provide the proper stability to your feet, especially when running on uneven surfaces.

Take the shoe, hold it by the heel with your right hand and the front with your left hand. Now twist the shoe in a motion that is similar to how you would squeeze water out of a cloth. Most runners want a shoe that does not flex too much. At the end of the day, you will be clocking up the miles in the running shoes, so pick something that will work for you.

Don't forget, if you are unsure; consult the professionals at the store where you are buying your shoes.

Choosing the correct shoes. Is cushioning needed?

Cushioning inside running shoes have become a very contentious subject of late. Some recent studies, most notably one conducted Medicine Research Laboratory in Luxembourg in 2013, have shown that these shoes do not result in fewer injuries than other types of running shoes.

The main reason for this that without all the extra padding, our feet are allowed to do what is expected of them while we run. They become less flexible, much stronger and adapts easily. The opposite happens with cushioned shoes. The foot is kept in place and can weaken over a long period. Whether you want cushioned shoes is down to personal preference at the end of the day.

The importance of running socks

The next most important piece of running equipment is your socks. You will run mile after mile in running socks, and they need to perform some important tasks. These include allowing your feet to breathe, remove moisture from your feet through wicking, help to maintain a cool temperature around your feet and finally and probably the most obvious, prevent your feet from blistering.

When choosing running socks, take the following into account.

- Fabric

  Many people who start out running will purchase a normal cotton sock, an easy mistake to make. Cotton is not the best fabric for a running sock as it firstly absorbs any sweat coming from the feet and secondly, it then holds that moisture. Wet socks are something all runners should avoid as it can lead to blisters.

  A perfect running sock can be made from a range of materials. These are almost always synthetic, including polyester and acrylic. If you find yourself running in very cold conditions, consider socks made from a wool blend. They will keep your feet warm while offering excellent moisture management.

- Thickness

  Often the thickness of a running sock is down to the individual runner but can be adjusted depending on the distance you will be running. A thinner sock can be used for runs over shorter distances while it is often beneficial to wear a thicker sock when running for long periods of time. Thicker socks can also help to keep your feet warm in colder conditions.

- Style

  Style is often down to personal preference but can depend on where you are running. If you are running on trails or through vegetation, consider knee-high socks for extra protection. They are also very useful for preventing loose stones from entering into your running shoes. Other options that are becoming popular are "toe" socks. They have sections for each toe on your foot.

- Size

  Always wear the correct size sock! If they are too big, they will move around in your running shoe. This friction can eventually lead to blisters. Socks that are too small can restrict blood flow and toe movement.

You might consider compression socks depending on how far you run each day. These socks are beneficial if you cover a lot of mileage as they gradually compress, increasing blood flow. They are extremely helpful in helping to reduce and even prevent shin splints and cramp. A word of warning, do not let the socks compress too much as you run.

Other important equipment

We have covered the essentials when it comes to running, but there are few other items that can make your running experience that much more enjoyable. Let's take a look at a few of them.

- Running vest and shorts

  Although these seem fairly obvious, it is very important to get the right running vest and shorts, especially if you want to be comfortable as you become fitter and begin to increase your mileage each session. Your clothing should be able to remove the sweat from your body as you run. This process, called "wicking", ensures that a runner feels more comfortable. Make sure your vest and shorts fit properly as well as this goes a long way to preventing chafing.

- Hat and sunglasses

  Whether you run with a hat and sunglasses comes down to personal preference. It is a great way to keep out the sun however, especially true when you are either running when it is rising or setting.

- Chafing stick/Lip protection/Sunscreen

  A must have accessory for those longer runs, a chafing stick can help to stop chafing in a number of areas. Proper sunscreen and lip balm application is also essential to protect your skin, even in overcast conditions.

- Storage belts

  These belts are useful for keeping your valuables safe during training sessions. Some are even able to carry small water bottles and energy gels. Again, these are a personal preference.

- Heart rate monitor/Watch

  These are very useful for measuring your heart rate as you run as well as the time you have exercised for.

Chapter 4 – Warm up routines

It is important to undertake a thorough warm up routine before you begin to run. Not only will the routine get your legs ready for the exercise ahead but more importantly, a warm up helps to increase the temperature of your muscles, allowing them to contract and relax easily as they workout.

An extensive warm up also helps to ensure proper blood circulation through the body, ensuring that oxygen is carried to each muscle efficiently, especially those used while running. Lastly, a warm up has mental benefits as well. It helps to focus our minds on the task ahead.

How to warm up properly

To ensure that you have warmed up correctly, try these easy exercises. They are perfect, whether you are running for 5km or 50km. The great thing about these warm up routines is that you only need around 20 metres of space in front of you to execute them properly.

- High Skips

  This exercise is similar to skipping but without a rope, although you are aiming to gain more height. As you jump upwards, concentrate on raising your knee in an upward motion on each jump. Start with your left leg and alternate as you proceed. You might need to use the opposite arm to help stabilise yourself, especially if you jump fairly high.

- Butt Kicks

  Slowly move forward in a straight line and starting with your left foot flick backwards so that your heel connects with your butt. Start off slowly, alternating between your left and right feet, building up speed as you go along until you are performing the warm up fairly quickly. Try to focus on making sure your heel strikes your butt on every kick.

- High Knees

  This exercise is an 180-degree reversal of the butt kick. Here you want to bring your needs up towards your chest, starting with your left foot and alternating as you move slowly forward. Again, you want to focus on achieving a fairly decent speed executing the exercise. Do not worry about how much distance you move forward. Repeat this 10 times for each leg.

- Walking lunges

  There are similar to a lunge except you will be walking forward slowly. Take a step with your left leg. Slowly began to lower your frame downwards. The object is to make an 90-degree angle between your left leg (the front) and your right leg (the back). When you do this correctly, your knee of your front leg will be straight over your ankle. Move slowly upwards and repeat but this time with your right leg. Do this 10 times in total.

- Frankenstein

  Place your arms out in front of you at 90 degrees to your body. Starting with your left leg, kick in an upwards motion. You need to aim to hit your palm of your left hand with your left toe, keeping your leg as straight as possible, and your toes pointed upwards. Alternate to your right leg. Do 15 kicks for each leg.

- Leg swings

  You will need something to support you when doing these exercises. Start by holding onto a wall with your right hand while beginning to swing your opposite leg. First swing forward, return to your starting position and then swing it backwards. Concentrate on making each swing a full motion without any pauses. Try and swing the leg as far forward or as far backwards as it can possibly go. Do 15 swings for each leg before changing to swinging each leg in a similar motion, but this time across the body.

What about stretching?

Although these warm up routines should be more than adequate to set you up for your run, some runners also like to incorporate a stretching routine before they run. Here are a few stretches that you can try. Repeat each of these three times. You will need a wall to perform some of them.

- Calf stretch

    Face the wall and place your arms out in front of you. Place your palms upwards against the wall while keeping your feet flat on the ground around a shoulder length apart. Now slowly lean forward with your hips. As you do this, start to bend your knees a little. You will begin to feel your calves stretch as you do this.

- Lower calf stretch

    Bend your body forward, keeping your palms in an upright position against the wall (your body should be roughly 90 degrees to the wall). Move your left foot forward and bend your knee slightly. Slowly lift your left foot upwards. You will begin to feel your lower calf stretch as you do this. Repeat with your right leg.

- Triceps and shoulder stretch

    Standing tall, take hold of your left elbow with your right hand. Begin to pull your elbow towards your body. You will feel your triceps and shoulder begin to stretch as you do this. Repeat with your right elbow.

- Hamstring stretch
  Stand upright, bend forward and touch your toes, moving up and down slowly by no more than 10 centimetres. You will begin to feel your hamstrings stretch as you do this.

- Quadriceps stretch

  Face the wall, stand on your right foot only using the wall to balance. Now hold your right foot with your left hand behind you. Begin to pull the foot towards your buttocks. You will begin to feel your quadriceps stretch as you do this. Repeat with your right leg.

- Groin stretch

  Sit on the ground and place your feet together but with the soles of your shoes touching each other. Now place your elbows on your knees and slowly begin to lean forward. Use your elbows to press your knees towards the ground. You will begin to feel your groin stretch as you do this.
  Now you are ready to tackle anything the road or trail can throw at you!

Chapter 5 – Running weight loss plan (8 weeks)

In this chapter, we will look at a running plan that will help you to lose weight. This plan will only work in conjunction with other factors that include:

- Healthy eating

  Losing weight is simple. You need to burn more calories than you consume. Running will go a long way to helping you burn those calories but this does not mean that you can eat whatever you like. Keep to a balanced, healthy diet ensuring that you include carbohydrates, protein, fat, minerals and vitamins in it. It is easy to fall into the trap of eating bigger portions (and, therefore, more food) to fuel our running. Try to keep to smaller meals and eat more regularly. Keeping a food journal is also a great way to see what you end up putting into your system. Do not skip meals as a way to save calories. Not eating properly will affect your running performance as your muscles will not have fuel to use to work effectively. For weight loss, you will need to burn 3500 calories to lose one pound of fat. There is no point in making your task more difficult by making bad food choices.

- Use a training plan

  A training plan is a great way to ensure that you train properly and keep your motivation levels up. A plan is of particular importance as it is designed to build towards a certain goal. Skipping a day, therefore, will set you back. We will be looking at an extensive training plan later in this chapter.

- Mix it up

  Although a training plan can be very specific, you can make slight changes as you run. Try incorporating interval training into your runs. Interval training does not require any extra running, just increase your speed for a period while you run. For example, run flat out for 30 seconds every five minutes, a great way to burn extra calories. Interval training can also raise your resting metabolic rate, burning more calories without exercise.

There are many examples of running plans that help you to lose weight. Often they included some form of strength training. This builds muscle, enabling them to burn even more calories. This plan incorporates some strength training as well.

Running plan workouts

This plan consists of four different types of training of which three incorporate running.

- Running to burn fat

  Here you will need to run at around 65% of your maximum heart rate. If you are unsure of what your maximum heart rate is, subtract your age from 220. For example, 220 − 45 (age) = 175. A heart rate in the region of 65% of this is around 113 beats per minute.

  If you do not have a heart rate monitor, run slightly faster than 50% of your full effort.

- Strength training

  There are a number of exercises that can be performed to build strength. The easiest of these to do without any additional equipment are push-ups, planks, squats and lunges. Consider joining a gym for strength training as well.

- Interval sprinting

  This run is specifically targeted at raising your heart rate and helping to burn extra calories. You will either need a treadmill set on an 8 percent incline or a hill on your favourite running route. Begin by running for 5 minutes at a relatively easy pace to warm up. Then sprint up the hill for 30 seconds followed by two minutes of recovery, either on a flat surface (on your treadmill or the road). Complete the number of hill sprints as indicate and finish with a 5 minute warm down.

- Relaxing run

  In this exercise, you will run for 20 minutes at a relaxed pace.

The running plan itself

This plan continues for 8 weeks. Remember, if you suffer from any health problems always consult your doctor before undertaking any new training regime.

56 DAY PROGRAM

Week 1

1 Monday: Run to burn fat: 15 minutes

2 Tuesday: Strength training: 10 minutes

3 Wednesday: Interval sprinting: 4 hill sprints (with a 5 minute
4 warm up & warm down).

4 Thursday: Rest or relaxing run: 20 minutes

5 Friday: Strength training: 10 minutes

6 Saturday: Run to burn fat: 20 minutes

7 Sunday: Rest

Week 2

8 Monday: Run to burn fat: 20 minutes

9 Tuesday: Strength training: 15 minutes

10 Wednesday: Interval sprinting: 5 hill sprints (with a 5 minute
warm up & warm down).

11 Thursday: Rest or relaxing run: 20 minutes

12 Friday: Strength training: 15 minutes

13 Saturday: Run to burn fat: 30 minutes

14 Sunday: Rest

Week 3

15 Monday: Run to burn fat: 25 minutes

16 Tuesday: Strength training: 20 minutes

17 Wednesday: Interval sprinting: 6 hill sprints (with a 5 minute warm up & warm down)

18 Thursday: Rest or relaxing run: 20 minutes

19 Friday: Strength training: 20 minutes

20 Saturday: Run to burn fat: 35 minutes

21 Sunday: Rest

Week 4

22 Monday: Run to burn fat: 20 minutes

23 Tuesday: Strength training: 15 minutes

24 Wednesday: Interval sprinting: 5 hill sprints (with a 5 minute warm up & warm down)

25 Thursday: Rest or relaxing run: 20 minutes

26 Friday: Strength training: 15 minutes

27 Saturday: Run to burn fat: 30 minutes

28 Sunday: Rest

Week 5

29 Monday: Run to burn fat: 25 minutes

30 Tuesday: Strength training: 20 minutes

31 Wednesday: Interval sprinting: 7 hill sprints (with a 5 minute warm up & warm down)

32 Thursday: Rest or relaxing run: 20 minutes

33 Friday: Strength training: 20 minutes

34 Saturday: Run to burn fat: 35 minutes

35 Sunday: Rest

Week 6

36 Monday: Run to burn fat: 30 minutes

37 Tuesday: Strength training: 25 minutes

38 Wednesday: Interval sprinting: 8 hill sprints (with a 5 minute warm up & warm down)

39 Thursday: Rest

40 Friday: Strength training: 25 minutes

41 Saturday: Run to burn fat: 40 minutes

42 Sunday: Rest

Week 7

43 Monday: Run to burn fat: 35 minutes

44 Tuesday: Strength training: 30 minutes

45 Wednesday: Interval sprinting: 9 hill sprints (with a 5 minute warm up & warm down)

46 Thursday: Rest or relaxing run: 20 minutes

47 Friday: Strength training: 30 minutes

48 Saturday: Run to burn fat: 45 minutes

49 Sunday: Rest

Week 8

50 Monday: Run to burn fat: 40 minutes

51 Tuesday: Strength training: 35 minutes

52 Wednesday: Interval sprinting: 10 hill sprints (with a 5 minute warm up & warm down)

53 Thursday: Rest or relaxing run: 20 minutes

54 Friday: Strength training: 35 minutes

55 Saturday: Run to burn fat: 50 minutes

56 Sunday: Rest

There you have it! It can be pretty tough but adjust as you need to. Good luck!

Chapter 6 – Post run warm downs

A proper warm down is often the last thing a runner thinks of after completing a gruelling session. Warming down in a proper manner is almost as important as your pre-run warm up.

Why are warm downs important?

A warm down routine helps the muscles, and the body for that matter, return to a normal state. Your heart rate, as well as your breathing, will slow down as your core body temperature drops. A proper cool down also performs the following very important functions.

- Stops blood from pooling

    While running, our muscles in our legs contract, sending blood back to our heart for it to once again pump it back through our bodies. If you just stop after completing a run, blood can begin to pool in your legs as your muscles have stopped contracting. This leads to a massive drop in blood pressure, dizziness or sometimes fainting, in very extreme cases. By cooling down your body resumes normal operation naturally.

- Helps to remove lactic acid build up

    While we exercise, lactic acid builds up in your muscles. By using a warming down routine, lactic acid is removed from the muscles.

- Reduces levels of adrenaline

    While running, the body releases adrenaline raising our heart rate, blood pressure and increasing our breathing rate. Warming down helps to remove this adrenaline from our system, thus helping with the body's recovery rate.

- Aids muscle recovery

    Lastly, by warming down properly, you allow your muscles to recover quicker, reducing the risk of injury in future running sessions.

How do you warm down properly?

While warming down you should consider drinking some form of energy supplement to replace the electrolytes lost while running.

Your warm down session can be as simple as slowing down your run to a slow pace or even a jog for at least the last two miles. You could even consider walking at a fast pace instead of running. Your body enters a recovery mode if you can keep your heart rate at around 70% of its maximum level.

Stretching is equally as important. After a run, your muscles are flexible, and stretching can help reduce the risk of injury. You can run through the warm up stretches from Chapter 4 to target all the important muscles that might need stretching. Hold each stretch for around 20 to 30 seconds, repeating at least twice for each muscle.

Chapter 7 – How to stay motivated

No matter how much we want to run, staying motivated over a long period of time can be difficult. The training plan in Chapter 5 is for eight weeks. That is the equivalent of two months and two months is a long time!

There are a number of ways to stay motivated, however. Remember, you are running to improve your fitness and lose weight! Let's look a few quick tips for staying motivated.

- Set goals

  At the beginning of the training plan, set yourself a weight loss goal. Don't let it be something unobtainable. Keep it realistic and within reach. You should have a fair idea of how much weight you think you can lose over the eight weeks. When you don't feel like running, remember your goal and what you want to achieve. Keep your eye on the prize!

- Get a running buddy

  Running with someone is a great way to stay motivated. On days that you do not feel like hitting the tarmac, a running buddy is often the motivation needed to get out there and do it anyway. The great thing is that this works both ways. On some days, you may need to motivate your running buddy!

- Try different running routes

  We all get bored with repetition, and the same goes for runners. Running the same route over and over again can become extremely boring, extremely quickly. Try a different route every week. You could even consider trading the tarmac for a nice trail run.

- Consider music

  Music is often a great way to take your mind off running down miles and miles of tarmac. Load up an MP3 player with your favourite tunes and watch the miles fly by!

- Treat yourself

  Another great motivator is to treat yourself for sticking to your goal. This could be something simple like a nice healthy meal at a local restaurant or even a long massage to ease those weary legs.

- Consider how lucky you are

  Many people that would like to run do not have the opportunity. Go out there and enjoy the chance you have been given.

Chapter 8 – Other considerations while training

There are a number of other aspects connected to running that you will need to consider each time you step outside your door in your running shoes.

Keep hydrated

As you run you begin to sweat, this expels important fluids out of your body, and it is essential that you replace these liquids. Let's take a look at a few tips for keeping hydrated while you run.

- Drink water along your route

  Either take water with you while you run or stop and drink water along the way. For every 20 minutes that you run try to drink around 200 to 300 milliliters of water. If you are running for a long period, you might consider a sports drink to help replace any electrolytes your body has lost. A word of warning, you can overhydrate. Listen to your body, muscles consist mostly of water. If you suddenly feel fatigued, the chances are your body needs water.

- Consider fruits

  A fruit is a great way to get some fluids into your body as well as important vitamins, minerals and electrolytes. Bananas, which are high in potassium, are a great fruit to eat while you run. Do not let a fruit replace water, however, you will still need to drink regularly.

- Weigh yourself before and after

  Weigh yourself before you begin your run and again straight after. If your weight drops by 3%, you might be dehydrated. Replacing water lost through exercise is just as important in the hours after the exercise is finished.

- Pay attention to your mouth

  Dehydration often manifests itself in the form of a dry mouth. If your mouth starts to get dry or parched, drink water immediately.

- Check your skin

  Another way to see if you are keeping your body hydrated is to pinch the fleshy skin near the back of your hand. If it returns into position fairly quickly your hydration levels are fine. If it takes some time, you might be starting to become dehydrated. Stop and drinks some water!

Safety

Keeping yourself safe while out running is of paramount importance. Follow these quick safety tips each time you leave for a training session.

- Tell someone where you will be running and for how long you plan to train.
- Keep a form of identification on your person when you run.
- Keep out of the road if possible.
- Always run towards traffic. You will be more visible and can see oncoming cars easier.
- Invest in high visibility clothing either in the form of a bib or a belt. This is especially necessary if you are running at dusk or dawn. If you run at night, consider a headlamp.
- If you do listen to music, keep the volume low so as to hear surrounding noises. Some runners often only run with one earpiece in their ears.
- Approach hills with caution, especially if you are running on the road. Sun glare can impair a driver's ability to see you.
- Don't run in areas that are not safe or are known to have heavy traffic.
- Obey the rules of the road like other pedestrians would.
- Do not run in isolated areas.
- Consider running with a friend.
- Consider running with a dog.

Chapter 9 – Running indoors

You might be lucky enough to either own a treadmill or have a gym membership and, therefore, have access to a treadmill.

Treadmills are a great way to continue your running plan, especially if the weather takes a turn for the worse. Running on a treadmill is very different to running on the open road, however. These handy tips can help you prepare for a run indoors.

- Be prepared

  This would appear to be pretty obvious, but once you have started on a treadmill you do not want to get off until your run is over. Make sure you have everything with you that you might need including water and a towel to wipe down, especially if you do not own the treadmill!

  Equipment wise, running on a treadmill is no different to running outside. Ensure you have the correct running clothes, socks and, of course, your running shoes.

- Don't forget to warm up

  Again, warming up correctly is just as important before a session on the treadmill as it is when running on the road. Perform your pre-run stretches and once you begin on the treadmill itself, start off slowly. Follow this great treadmill warm up - walk for 3 minutes, jog for 3 minutes and then ease into a run, increasing the speed slowly until you reach a comfortable level.

- Use the incline

  One advantage of a treadmill is that it can simulate hills whenever you want; great for the incline running section of our training plan in Chapter 5. Running up an incline is also an excellent way to get your heart rate up and to burn more calories!

- Don't forget to warm down

  A proper warm down is just as important as your warm up. Many people use this simple equation to warm down after a treadmill run. Walk on the treadmill for 1 minute for every mile you have covered during your run. Don't forget to stretch afterward.

Chapter 10 - Five quick weight loss tips for runners

Finally, let's look at five quick weight loss tips that will further supplement the training plan from Chapter 5.

- Aim for a small calorie deficit

  By eating around 300 to 500 calories less per day, you can aid your weight loss. Do not cut your calories more than this. Your body will still need fuel while training, so this can be a tricky balancing act.

- Strength training is important

  Try not to skip the strength training. This form of exercise is not everybody's favourite, but it does help to build muscle that leads to an increased metabolism allowing your body to burn fat even while resting. Stronger muscles mean fewer injuries, another added benefit.

- The importance of interval sprinting

  Interval sprinting (which forms part of the training plan) is an excellent way to burn fat and, therefore, lose weight.

- The importance of protein

  There is much debate currently about Low Carb diets and increased protein intake. Firstly, protein can keep you feeling fuller for longer and secondly, it works hand in hand with strength training to help build muscle.

Conclusion

Thank you very much for purchasing this book!

It gives you the necessary information to use running to help you lose weight. Use this knowledge, apply it and over the course of 8 weeks, you will not only be much fitter, but you will have lost weight!

This book, however, is filled with so much more interesting information, all beneficial to those of you that pound the tarmac day in and day out.

Lastly, remember, before you undertake any change in training regime, you should consult your doctor.

Printed in Great Britain
by Amazon